Teaching Adults to Swim

*Dedicated to my family: my wife Renee—my raison d'être,*
*and my family: Travis, Sara, and Danielle, and*
*newest swim students—grandsons Sawyer and Noah*

Brian "Flash" Fagan

# TEACHING ADULTS TO
# SWIM
## USING THE FLASH AQUATIC SWIM TECHNIQUE

## The Perfect Guide for Swim Instructors

Meyer & Meyer Sport

British Library Cataloguing in Publication Data
A catalogue record for this book is available from the British Library

**Teaching Adults to Swim**
Maidenhead: Meyer & Meyer Sport (UK) Ltd., 2025
ISBN: 978-1-78255-282-6

All rights reserved, especially the right to copy and distribute, including the translation rights.
No part of this work may be reproduced–including by photocopy, microfilm or any other
means–processed, stored electronically, copied or distributed in any form whatsoever without
the written permission of the publisher.

© 2025 by Meyer & Meyer Sport (UK) Ltd.
Aachen, Auckland, Beirut, Cairo, Cape Town, Dubai, Hägendorf, Hong Kong, Indianapolis,
Maidenhead, Manila, New Delhi, Singapore, Sydney, Tehran, Vienna

Member of the World Sport Publishers' Association (WSPA), www.w-s-p-a.org

Printed by King Printing Company, Inc., Lowell, MA
www.kingprinting.com
Printed in the United States of America

ISBN 978-1-78255-282-6
Email: info@m-m-sports.com
www.thesportspublisher.com

Manufacturer under the GPSR
Meyer & Meyer Fachverlag und Buchhandel GmbH
Von-Coels-Str. 390
52080 Aachen, Germany
www.dersportverlag.de

Beginner students should only swim in the presence of a certified swim instructor.
The content of this book was carefully researched. However, readers should always consult
a qualified medical specialist for individual advice before adopting any new exercise plan.
This book should not be used as an alternative to seeking specialist medical advice.

All information is supplied without liability. Neither the author nor the publisher will be
liable for possible disadvantages, injuries, or damages.

# CONTENTS

# ACKNOWLEDGMENTS

I would like to acknowledge the following people who helped in the development of *Teaching Adults to Swim* and to those who helped in turning this book into a reality.

Mary Strevel for editing my first draft and turning it into a book.

Richard Karossy for the photography both above and underwater, and to Renee Fagan as my swim student model.

My managing editor, Liz Evans, at Meyer & Meyer, for her tremendous help with this book from beginning to end.

Mike Lazzara and Chris Dunn of the Rutherford Swim Association for believing in me and giving me a facility in which *Teaching Adults to Swim* was born and nurtured into the reality it is today. Thanks guys! Mike, no truer words were ever spoken than when we first met, and you said: "I want you to consider this your home." Chris, thanks for your help with additional photography. To Diane Wojcik for all her help with scheduling.

Last and foremost to my age group and high school swim coach and mentor: Charles M. Schlegel. Except for my father, no man had a stronger influence in shaping the person I am today and who taught me that with hard work, dedication, and perseverance anything was possible. He also showed me first-hand the joy and rewards that came from teaching and coaching. Coach Schlegel would say: "Bring the swimmer to me when they are young, and they are mine for life." Thanks, Coach.

# INTRODUCTION

I have always been passionate about swimming; swimming saved my life.

As an infant I had life-threatening asthma, which often resulted in hospitalization and time in an oxygen tent. During one of those visits, a doctor suggested to my parents that learning to swim might build up my lung power. I was five at the time, and my parents immediately enrolled me into swimming lessons at the YMCA in Flushing, Queens, New York.

The YMCA had and still has an excellent swim instruction program for young people. I took to swim lessons right away and quickly went through the various age group swim badges and, before long, became a member of the Y's competitive swim team.

Hello swim team, and goodbye inhalers and oxygen tents. I continued to work hard at swimming, eventually becoming a New York State swim champion and a division II collegiate swimmer.

Swimming also led me to lifeguard certification (surely one of the best and most rewarding jobs for a young person) and becoming an ocean lifeguard at Jones Beach and Robert Moses State Park for 13 years.

Swimming has been so fulfilling in my life that I wanted to share it with others, and have dedicated myself to teaching others how to swim.

What you are about to read is the result of those decades spent working with swim students and the culmination of what worked best with students and what did not.

I became increasingly disenchanted with traditional swim teaching methods for adults—with their immediate focus on floating and breathing.

To my mind, beginning swim lessons with breathing and floating was like trying to teach someone how to ride a bicycle by starting them with a unicycle!

One of the key elements that was missing from conventional teaching was showing the student how to stand in the water. Many adult beginners, if not most, have the fear: "Once I start moving in the water, will I be able to stand up again?" They literally had to learn **to stand before they could swim**.

Additionally, showing someone how to stand in the water was neither intuitive nor simply conveyed. There were a series of moves that had to be taught, demonstrated, and synchronized to achieve the standing motion.

Once the student was able to do these moves and stand with ease, much of their fear dropped away and their progress accelerated dramatically. Many of my students, once the standing had been mastered, were swimming in just one lesson—with complete waterproofing coming in just a few sessions. When I say "waterproofing," I mean the ability to jump into the deep end of the pool, come up and tread water, and then swim a length of the pool. Something that only less than 25% of the adult population in America can do!

When I had students tell me they had taken swimming lessons multiple times and had never been taught my method or experienced such rapid progress, I realized I was on to something that had to be shared with coaches and nonswimmers. This book is the result.

There is a drowning epidemic in this country. Fatal drowning is the leading cause of death for children ages 1-4 and the second leading cause of death for ages 5-14. I believe this is a systemic problem, with adults who do not know how to swim being more likely to have children who do not know how to swim. Once an adult learns how to swim, they are more comfortable seeking out swimming environments as a family and will encourage their children to take swim lessons if they do not already know how to swim.

Consequently, it is of vital importance that adults are taught how to swim, and this book can be instrumental in achieving that goal.

Remember that we will be teaching the students what works best to become swimmers, rather than the refined techniques of a competitive swimmer—that will come later.

They say that when the student is ready, the teacher will appear. I am here, and you are ready.

Let us begin.

# PART I
# TEACHING FREESTYLE

## Section 1
## Overview/The Interview

The purpose of the overview is to acquaint your students with what they can expect from your lesson plan. The overview also puts the students at ease when they know that the lessons will be tailored to suit and address their overall comfort level in the water.

Explain to the student that the main factor with the lessons is that they are always comfortable, and that they find the experience rewarding and have fun with it.

Now explain the lesson plan to the student and what steps will be taken over time. It is important to stress to the student that the pace of the lessons will be based on their comfort level, how fast they can adapt to the lessons, and whether they are fearful or phobic about the water and the level of that distress. All nonswimmers are afraid of the water to some degree, and rightly so—they do not know how to swim and unassisted could drown—not an unreasonable concern.

Tell the swimmer that by the end of the lessons, they will be what you consider to be "waterproof," that is, able to jump into the deep water, come to the surface, tread water, and then swim 25 yards. This will sound unbelievable to your swimmer, and the prospect of, at some point, jumping into deep water will be terrifying. Stress to the swimmer that all of this is a gradual process and will not happen until they are ready.

The student will want to know how long that takes. Tell them that every student is different, depending on their initial level of comfort, to what extent they may or may not be phobic in the water, and to what degree they are initially buoyant—the most crucial factor. Advise the student that a nonphobic or moderately phobic individual with adequate-to-good buoyance can usually achieve this in 10 lessons or about 10 hours.

Then explain that the further intent is to continue to work on their technique so that they can swim laps and use swimming as a workout for life—exercising the whole body with low impact.

It should also be explained to the student that they can learn other strokes as well—backstroke and breaststroke, and, if they are ambitious, the butterfly. Tell the student that additional strokes will expand how they can work out in the pool.

Now begins the interview process. An important part of the interview process is to inquire if your swimmer has any physical limitations that may prevent them from taking a full stroke. If that is the case—shoulder injury, for example—you will have to stay mindful of that in your teaching and advise the student you will work within their parameters.

During the interview process, you will also take their history regarding swim lessons—have they had any swim lessons or are they complete beginners. If they have had lessons, you may have to undo bad habits or techniques.

Also, during the interview process you will want to ascertain whether the student experienced any past trauma—did a family member throw them into the water? Any near-drowning incidents? Any traumatic incidents will almost certainly result in water phobia, and you will have to proceed cautiously.

A lack of past trauma is not always indicative of the swimmer being fearful. A student can still be extremely fearful without a history of near-drowning or bad experiences. It may not come up in the interview, even if you ask directly, "Are you afraid of the water." It may only become apparent once they are in the water, and putting their face in the water also may not elicit a strong response. The reaction will appear when you ask them to push off the wall, even slightly. If, after the smallest push-off, they come up grasping for support, you will know you are dealing with a fearful student and must move forward accordingly—(see section 8C, Dealing With the Fearful Swimmer).

Once the interview process is over, it is time to begin the lesson in the water.

# Section 2
# Making the Swimmer Comfortable in the Water

## A  Head Bobs

Help your swimmer adjust their goggles. Once the goggles are in place, have your swimmer put their face in the water and make sure there is no leakage. Hold your student's hands and tell them you are going to do head bobs, which are like underwater squats. Tell the student that they will be holding their breath for the first few head bobs.

Holding on to their hands and doing the drill with them, begin the head bobs by having the student drop below the surface, in a squat-like manner, taking a breath and holding it as they squat under the water with their head fully submerged. If your swimmer successfully executes the head bob, that is, they go straight down and the water is above their head, have them do it three or four times—all while holding their breath.

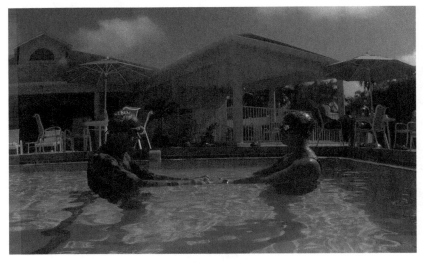

*Pre-head bob*

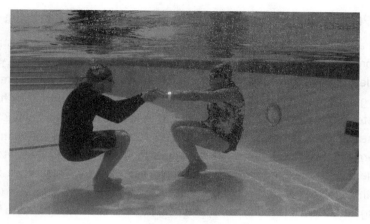

*Head bob—holding breath.*

## B  Heads Bobs With Exhaling

Tell the swimmer that they will now have to exhale their breath, which is done by blowing bubbles through their lips. Take the student's hand and blow softly into their palm. Now have the swimmer do several head bobs while exhaling, again holding their hands and doing it with them. Check that bubbles are coming out of their mouth and that they are fully exhaling.

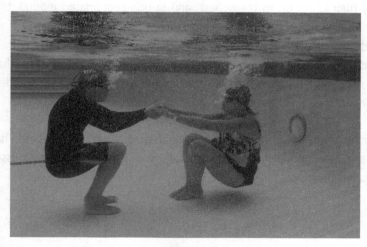

*Head bob—exhaling.*

## C  Push-Off and Stand—You Have to Stand Before You Can Swim

Just as you must stand before you can walk, a student must learn to stand before they can start swimming. Although it may seem counterintuitive, your student will not know how to stand up in the water once their feet are off the ground, and they will not be comfortable in the water until they have mastered this procedure. Tell the student that the movement to stand is the same as if they were stretched out in a chaise lounge chair and they want to return to a seated position—that is, to draw their arms to their chest at the same time as they pull their knees to their chest, and then plant their feet on the floor. Stress to the student that it is especially important that they bring both of their feet down at the same time, as it is extremely hard to find your balance with one foot and will cause them to stumble forward and lose their balance.

To help with this procedure, we will have the student use a "water barbell." The student will stand in the water next to the pool wall, and holding the barbell out in front of them, bring their feet up onto the pool wall and take a small push off from the wall with their face in the water—just a foot or two forward—and then bring the barbell to their chest at the same time they bring their knees up to their chest, and in one coordinated motion, bring their head up as they plant their feet down on the floor of the pool and stand up. Practice this movement until the student is comfortable with the standing motion. Stress to the student that they must start to lift their head up as soon as they are in motion. You will be surprised how many students do not lift their head out of the water.

Learning to stand will vary based on overall fitness and coordination. I have had some students pick it up immediately, while others take several lessons to master the process.

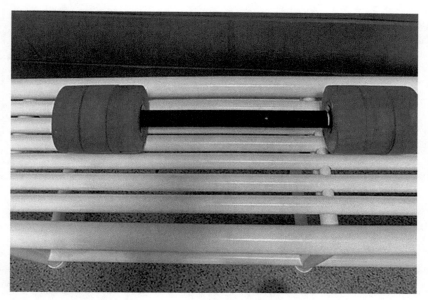

*Water barbell.*

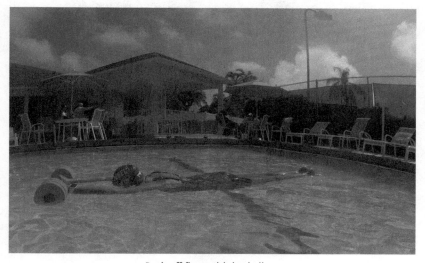

*Push-off float with barbell.*

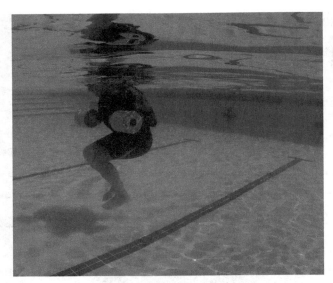

*Barbell—knees to chest.*

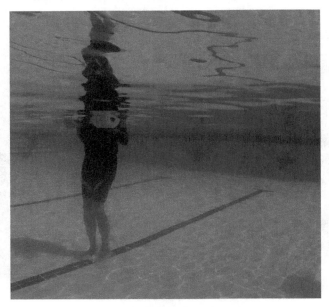

*Barbell—feet planted.*

# Section 3
# Superman/Superwoman Glide—
# With and Without Barbell

This is an easy move and the first indication of how buoyant your student is, how fast your lessons will proceed, and it will determine the future of your lesson plan. Tell your students that they are now going to do what you call the "Superman/Superwoman Glide."

Using the water barbell, have the swimmer push off the wall and glide on top of the water with their arms extended in front of them, their face in the water, and with the water level just below their hairline with their head looking along the lane marker on the pool floor, going as far as they are comfortable. Then have them execute the standing motion with the barbell. Demonstrate to the student the movement and tell them to take a breath and exhale in the water. When the student is comfortable with the glide and stand, have them try the glide without the barbell.

When the movement is completed with and without the barbell, it is time to introduce the kick.

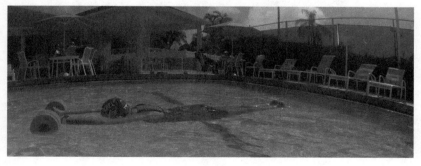

*Superwoman glide—no kick.*

# Section 4
# Gliding and Kicking—With and Without Barbell

To demonstrate the kick, have the swimmer hold on to the side of the pool and slowly bring their feet up. Grasp their ankles and demonstrate the proper kicking technique: keeping the legs straight, not bending the knees, and kicking down and up, just a few inches below the surface. Stress that the upward kick is as important as the downward. Make sure they do not bend their knees too much.

After demonstrating the proper kick movement, have the student push off from the wall with the barbell and glide and kick. Correct any faults they have with the kicking motion.

Once the student is comfortable with the glide, kick, and stand, have them try the movement without the barbell.

When doing the gliding movements without the barbell, be prepared that your swimmer may be very timid or fearful without the barbell to assist them. This is a big step for your student, and progress may be slow and require a great deal of patience on your part.

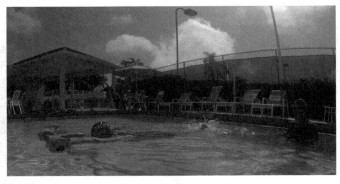

*Superwoman glide with kick.*

# Section 5
# Gliding and Kicking With Arms

While standing in the water and bending at the waist, demonstrate the arm motion, showing the student how to lift their elbows high and stretch out their arms, entering the water with their hands slightly cupped and their fingers pointing at a downward angle. I tell my students to picture trying to bring their elbows to the far wall before their hand enters the water.

Once the hand enters the water, the student will be executing what is called "the catch," which is where the cupped hand begins to move downward and catches the water. The arm pulls the water downward. This is the first part of the two-part action—the first part is the pull, where the hand pulls the water downward, and the second part, the push, is where the hand and arm pull the water backward until the hand is parallel with the hip. As the arm is pulling toward the hip, there is a slight bending and flaring out of the elbow. Without the elbow flair-out, shoulder problems may occur. And if both arms are not continually moving, the body will drag in the water.

Tell the student that it is especially important that both arms are in continuous motion—one arm is pulling downward while the other arm is lifting out of the water and moving into the catch position. If both arms are not continuously moving, it will result in the body dragging in the water.

Now have the swimmer try the glide while kicking and using their arms. Advise the student that they should imagine that they have an iron bar running through their shoulder blades and that bar is pressing them slightly down on the water, which will allow their butt and legs to come to the surface, making their body more streamline, which makes it easier to kick. At the same time, they should keep their torso in place and make sure they are not rolling that part of their body.

Correct any arm problems you observe. The most common problems are not lifting the elbows high enough and not doing a strong pull-down and really engaging the catch and pull action. They are, in effect, just "pawing" at the water and doing a shallow catch, which will not generate a strong pull–push and create an effective forward motion.

Another common problem, which goes along with "pawing" the water, is moving the arms too fast. This is a good time to demonstrate to your student the difference between a good swimmer and someone who is not swimming effectively, in other words, how the poor swimmer moves too fast, flays their arms, and splashes tremendously. Then show the smooth stroking and how it is splash-less. Demonstrating the "poor swimmer" will almost always get a laugh out of your student and is a great tension breaker!

Also check if your swimmer is listing to one side when they stroke. This indicates that the arm on the side they are moving toward is working harder than the other side. Tell the swimmer to be mindful to do a stronger pull–push with the other arm and see if their path is now straight.

It is important to note at this point whether your initial interview revealed that your student has had any shoulder problems. If they have had shoulder problems, the high elbow technique may prove painful or make it difficult for the swimmer to do the motion effectively and, at this point, it is advisable to have the swimmer do a sling movement with their arm—slinging their arm over the water rather than lifting their elbow and reaching forward. If your swimmer also has a natural inclination to doing a sling motion over the high elbow, you may want to stay with the sling movement.

This brings up a point to always keep in mind: **Do not sacrifice the good in pursuit of perfection**.

During this process, it is a good time to start filming what the student is doing. I have found that once students see what they are doing wrong, it makes things much easier to convey and correct.

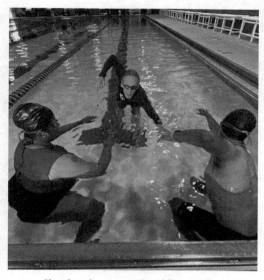

*Showing the arm stroke while standing.*

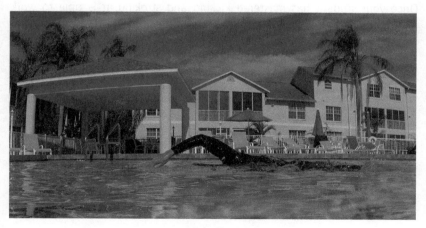

*High elbow.*

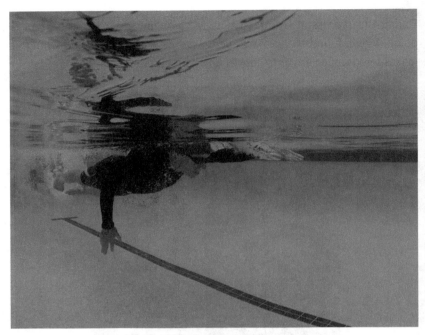

*Left arm catching and right arm pushing underwater.*

Once your student has mastered kicking and stroking, it is time to work on breathing.

# Section 6
# Breathing

Proper technique with breathing is one of the most, if not the most, important elements when learning to swim—particularly regarding the freestyle.

I tell my students that when someone is struggling with their freestyle, even as an experienced swimmer, either in the execution or with stamina, it is almost always rooted in difficulty with breathing and not using the proper breathing form.

First, we need to demonstrate how to take a breath. I like to tell my students to picture that they have a straw in the corner of their mouth, and they are taking a sip of air through that straw. The student then exhales that sip of air through their compressed lips by blowing bubbles—just as they did with head bobs. Tell the student that it is just a two- or three-beat inhalation and exhalation. A longer breath will be difficult to fully exhale.

Demonstrate and then have them do it with their face in the water. Once they can take a breath and exhale effectively, it is time to teach the head turn.

## A   Head Turn

The head turn is another key element in swimming. Efficiency in the water, or lack of, is very much dependent on a crisp, short head turn.

While standing, demonstrate by putting your face in the water, and tell them that half of their face remains in the water while one half of the face does the turn to get that "sip" of air. The head then returns to the center, and the breath is exhaled. Tell your swimmer to count—one-two, when taking the breath, and one-two, when they put their face back in the water to exhale. Have your swimmer practice the head turn and breathing while standing. When the swimmer is comfortable doing the head turn, it is time to synchronize the head turn with the arm motion and kicking.

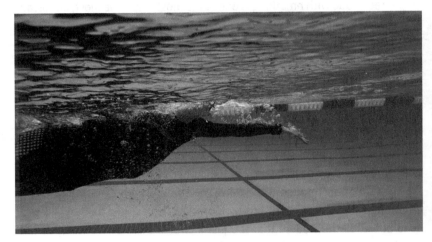

*Head turn.*

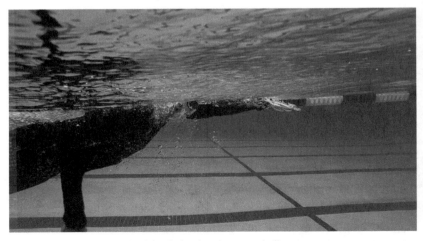

*Completing head turn—exhaling.*

## B   Head Turn With Arms

When synchronizing the arms with the breathing, it is important to stress to the swimmer that the head turn and breath must be executed when the lead arm is fully extended—that will be when a pocket of air is created. If the head turn is attempted when the lead arm is not fully extended, the body will be lower in the water. To get a breath would necessitate having to lift out of the water and raise the torso up to breathe. Proper breathing is when the lead arm is fully extended and the trailing arm is lifting out of the water with a high elbow. If the swimmer is turning their head to the right, they breathe when the left arm is fully extended. Should they breathe on their left side, the right arm must be fully extended. Have the student practice the arm stroking while standing.

While pushing off from the wall and kicking, have the swimmer take a few strokes, try to take one clean breath, and then take a few more strokes. Watch the swimmer as they take the breath—is the lead arm fully extended? How is their arm tempo—moving too fast or slow? Are their arms synchronized? Are they fully extending their arms and not letting their arms "catch-up" with each other? Check they getting a good pull–push with their strokes, or are they just "pawing" the surface? One of the key elements is making sure they are taking that "sip" of air.

When the swimmer is getting a clean first breath, you can have them try to take additional breaths.

Stress to the swimmer that one of the biggest problems with the breath is waiting too long to take it, which results in taking a big, "gasping" breath, which cannot be done with a slight head turn and will cause the swimmer to overcorrect and raise their torso out of the water and slow, if not completely arrest, forward momentum.

Once your swimmer has mastered three breaths, point out to them that they are now swimming! This is a real milestone for your student, so be sure to give it the importance that it deserves.

Point out to the swimmer that as they are now swimming above the water, it does not matter whether the pool depth is just a few feet or 10 feet deep— they are swimming on top of the water.

It is now time to begin the "waterproofing" process and teach the student how to float and tread water.

# Section 7
# The Final Frontier—Waterproofing

## A Back Float

Most swimmers find the back float an easy action to master, but that is not always the case, as even swimmers who have good buoyancy may struggle.

The maneuver is a simple one—the swimmer slowly leans back into the water by putting their head all the way back, chin pointed at the ceiling. Help the swimmer by tilting their head backward as you tell them to throw their shoulders back and bow their back while bringing their legs up. It may be helpful to position your hand in the small of the student's back while tilting their head. Tell the swimmer to spread their arms and legs into the starfish position.

Remove your hand and see if the swimmer can retain the floating position, even for just a few seconds. The student may find it helpful to slightly move their arms and legs.

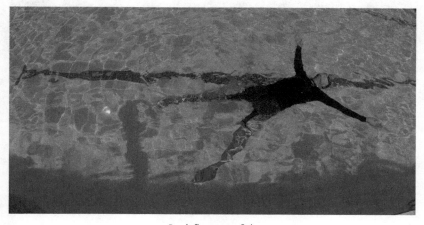

*Back float—starfish.*

## B   Back Float to Freestyle

Going from the back float to freestyle is an easy maneuver for most swimmers. When the swimmer is in the back float position, tell them to forcefully throw one arm across their chest while the other arm moves behind their back. This action will flip them onto their stomach, where they should begin to kick their feet and move their arms. It is important to stress to the student that it will take a while to work up forward momentum, and they must stay with it. When the student has mastered this action, remind them that it is one of the key ingredients in becoming waterproof. Whenever they are swimming and become tired, they can flip onto their back and rest and then resume swimming when they are ready.

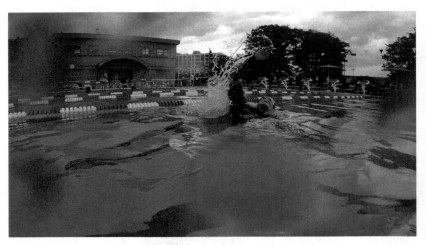

*Back float—arm throw over.*

## C  Treading Water

There are few elements more important for making a swimmer "waterproof" than treading water. It is also one of the most difficult aspects to teach.

Part of the difficulty with learning to tread water is that it involves two very different movements. The top action with the hands, which some people call "sculling," is hard to convey. You can tell the student to press the water down, away from the body, and then up, toward the body. Tell them to push the water out in such a way that the shoulder blades and the head come up out of the water.

Another guide is to tell them to picture making figure 8s in the water. Another good analogy is the word "sculling"—which is the action an oar in a rowboat makes when just grabbing the top of the water to propel the boat forward. The swimmer will tend to move their arms too frantically and will have to be told to slow down their action and relax.

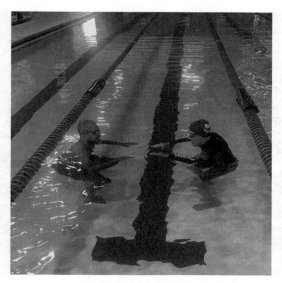

*Teaching sculling.*

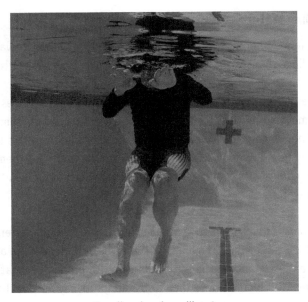

*Treading, hands sculling 1.*

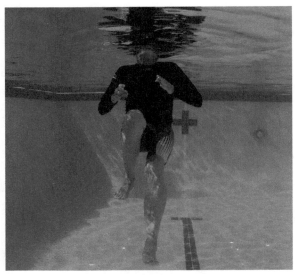

*Treading, hands sculling 2.*

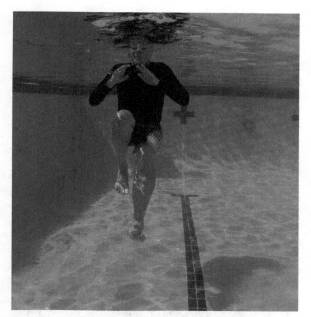

*Treading, hands sculling 3.*

The second part is to teach the kick. There are two different options when it comes to kicking. One option is a bicycle-like motion where the legs do a cycling, piston-like motion, bringing their knee up to their chest and continuously moving their legs. The best example to give the student is that of someone pedaling a bicycle. The second option is to have the swimmer move their legs from side to side. This kicking movement is known as "the eggbeater." Have the swimmer try both ways of kicking and see which they prefer. Most swimmers will gravitate to one type or the other. It may be helpful to have the swimmer lean back into a half back float position. Additionally, you may want to hold up the swimmer in the leaning back position, with a hand under the armpit and the other hand at the small of their back, and then release them, and see if they can manage to get their feet off the pool for a few seconds.

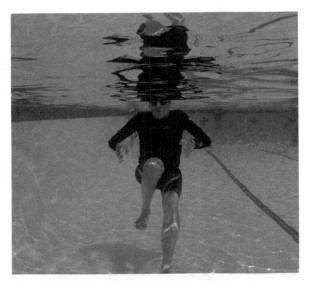

*Treading—bicycle kick 1.*

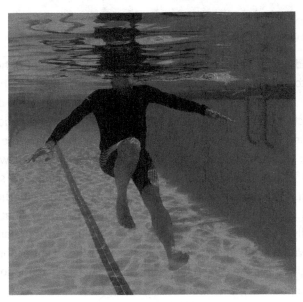

*Treading—bicycle kick 2.*

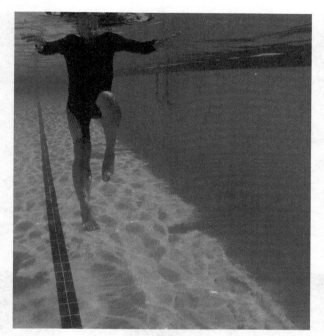

*Treading—bicycle kick 3.*

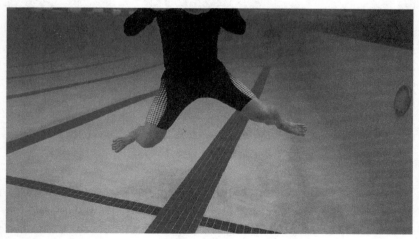

*Egg beater kick 1.*

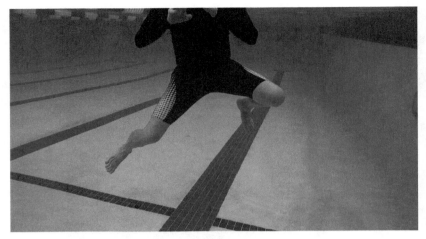

*Egg beater kick 2.*

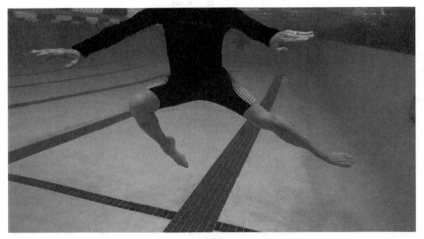

*Egg beater kick 3.*

The swimmer will likely move too quickly with both actions and must be reminded to slow down. Demonstrate to them a swimmer who is doing the actions too quickly and how tiring and ineffective that action is, and then demonstrate the proper movement and how little energy is being expended.

Tell the swimmer that the initial intent is to just get a few seconds with their feet off the floor and gradually increase the amount of time they are treading water. Congratulate and encourage the swimmer when they can increase their time treading. Success with treading water will vary greatly. Some students pick it up like magic, while others may struggle to master the movement through several classes. Body type is no indication of how a swimmer will fare with treading water; slender people with no body fat can struggle with treading, but that is not always the case.

Once your swimmer is comfortable with treading and can do it easily for several minutes, it is time to teach the treading to freestyle action.

## D   From Treading Water to Freestyle

Having your swimmer able to transition from treading to freestyle is the final element in being waterproof.

When the student is in the treading position, have them pull their arms to their chest, like the beginning of the standing motion, and at the same time, swing their legs out behind them with their legs together. This will put the swimmer on their stomach and in a prone position. Tell them that from there, they must start a strong kicking action and begin to move their arms. Let the swimmer know that, in this instance, it is okay to start with their head above water, but as soon as possible, they should put their face in the water. Stress to the swimmer, as with the back float to swimming, it is not an easy move to get their forward momentum going and they must stay with it.

Once the swimmer has mastered the movement, take a moment to acknowledge their achievement—they are now waterproof. Emphasize to the swimmer that they now have two movements they can do: the back float and treading, which they can use if they swallow water or if they get tired and need a moment to catch their breath or rest before continuing to swim.

Now comes the last part of waterproofing—deep water work.

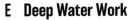
# E  Deep Water Work

### 1  Swimming in Deep Water

We have told the swimmer that once they are swimming on top of the water, it does not matter how deep the water is, and now it is time to prove that to the student.

Take them to the deep end of the pool, and have them slip into the water and hold on to the side of the pool, a lane or two from the end of the pool. Be in the water with the student, and have them push off and swim the corner section to the other side of the pool. This part will probably take a lot of encouragement. Once they have swum the corner, give the student a great deal of praise—this is a major milestone for them! Have the student repeat this action several times. When they are comfortable swimming the corner, have them push off from an end lane and swim out, taking two or three breaths, and then hold on to the side of pool.

It is now time to teach the student how to jump into deep water.

### 2  Jumping Into Deep Water

The technique I recommend for the student's first jump into the water is the same as how a lifeguard enters the water for a shallow rescue entry—legs are split, and their arms slap the water upon entry, with splayed legs that quickly jackknife together after entering the water. This will keep the swimmer from sinking too far down.

You will be in the water waiting for them with a lifeguard buoy. The student will be extremely nervous before their first jump—encourage them and let them know: "You got this." Demonstrate how they should enter the water, and then wait for them with the buoy. They will probably pace back and forth and need strong encouragement to take the first jump. Remind them that after entering the water, they will have to kick their legs and stroke their arms upward. **It is also advisable at this point for you to drop below the surface as they enter the water and make sure they are doing the motions to come to the surface. Be prepared for the fact that you may have to assist them to the surface.** When they do come to the surface, have them tread water. After a few tries with the shallow jump, have the student take a full jump in with their arms at their side. It is now particularly important to let them know that they will sink deeper in the water and will have to kick and stroke their arms more to rise to the surface. **Also be mindful that the depth to which your swimmer goes down below the surface may vary greatly.**

### 3   Jump In, Tread, Lap Swim

When the swimmer is comfortable with the jumping in and treading, it is time to have them try to swim a lap. Have them jump in, come to the surface, tread for a minute, and then push off from the wall and begin to swim. Tell the swimmer it does not matter how many times they have to stop and tread water or even hold on to the side of the pool, but you want them to swim a full lap. You will be alongside the swimmer with the buoy for encouragement and assistance as needed. This is also a good time to have someone video them as they do the lap because they will want a record of this achievement.

When your swimmer finishes the lap, be sure to let them know that they are now waterproof and able to do something that less than 25% of the United States population can do—swim the length of a pool! They are now a swimmer!

### 4   Jump In, Tread, Orient, and Exit Pool

Now that the swimmer has jumped in and swum a lap, they are usually eager to repeat the jumping-in process, so encourage that as much as possible, and as many times as they want to do it. You can also see if they want to try jumping off the pool starting blocks, if your pool has them.

This procedure may require the assistance of another instructor to help them get onto the blocks and make sure they are steady.

Once again, be in the water with a lifeguard buoy and be prepared for them to sink lower in the water (explain that fact to your student) and to go under with them.

Instruct the swimmer that when they come to the surface, they should do a treading motion that turns them around as they look for a swim ladder to use to exit the pool. Remind the student that this is the procedure they will use to exit a pool and that they should always be mindful of where the pool exits are.

# Section 8
# Problem-Solving—The Buoyance Paradox

## A  Sinkers

One of the most difficult areas of teaching swimming is dealing with students who have little or no buoyancy. One of the strangest aspects in dealing with buoyancy is that people with higher body fat often have better buoyancy than those with little or no body fat—which can be extremely frustrating for someone with little or no body fat. *I'm a conditioned athlete, why is this happening to me?* Their frustration will be increased by the fact that they have been able to excel in other sports and athletic events, so why are they struggling with swimming? Additionally mystifying is the fact that this is not always the case with low body fat. There are lean swimmers who immediately take to treading water without a problem. There are also swimmers who take to treading water right away but have difficulty with back floating and vice versa. You will be unable to tell how well someone does with treading water or back floating until they try it.

A distinction must be made between swimmers who have trouble staying above water when trying to tread and those who immediately start to sink.

With a student who manages a moment or two above the water before dropping under, it is just a matter of having them stay with it until they become more comfortable with treading. It is quite common for the student to be moving too quickly with the treading motion and taking their arms too wide or not pressing down enough to lift their body out of the water.

This is very different from the student who cannot manage even a few seconds on top of the water and immediately starts to sink and, indeed, looks very much like a drowning person. (Ironically, students who are very fit and have well developed abs are likely to fall into this category as their middle section will be very dense).

You will have to proceed slowly with the student prone to sinking. Have the student practice win-sprints in the shallow end, running and lifting their knees high. The next step is to have them practice the treading motions while wearing a waist aqua belt or a life jacket. While wearing them yourself, demonstrate the treading motion.

Wearing the belt or jacket should alleviate the student's stress level in attempting to tread. Once the student appears comfortable doing the treading motions while wearing the gear, remove it and see how they do without it. The intent now, as with the unfearful student, is to get a few seconds with their feet off the ground. Hopefully, the student is now able to perform even a rudimentary version of treading. If they still cannot manage it, you will have to repeat the training with the gear until they are comfortable.

There is also the stark reality that some students are physiologically incapable of treading, and try as they might, cannot manage more than a few seconds of treading, which will not be enough to help them catch their breath when swallowing water or being able to see an exit point after jumping into the water.

Once again, this calls for flexibility on the part of the instructor. I have found that with students who fall into this class, it is helpful to replace treading with a hybrid mix of breaststroke and a "doggie paddle"—any combination of movements that will allow the student to stay in place long enough to catch their breath and/or be able to find an exit route.

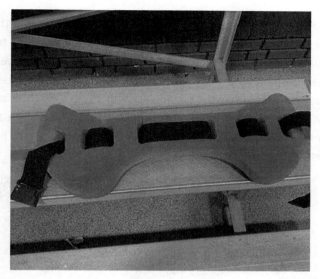

*Waist aqua belt.*

# B  Lower Body Draggers

Another buoyancy problem is with swimmers prone to lower body drag, that is, their waist, hips, and legs are too low in the water. Lower body drag creates a host of stroke problems: lack of forward momentum, reduced stamina, and the upper body has to raise out of the water to take a breath.

The root cause of lower body drag is usually due to the swimmer positioning their head too high and an ineffective kick. Remind the swimmer of the iron bar running across their shoulder blades and to press down on that bar, which will cause their lower body to come up. Also, with this problem, it is recommended that the student swims with their head lower in the water than is usually recommended.

Tell the swimmer that they will have to work on a strong kick to help compensate for their body drag. It is also advisable to break the "stiff leg" kicking rule and tell the swimmer that some amount of knee bend will be okay. Also advise the swimmer to drop their head lower than the usual below-the-hairline standard. Have the student use a pull buoy and tell them that it puts their lower body into the position it should naturally be in. This lower head position may make a quick head turn difficult, so observe the student as they take a breath and work with them accordingly. It may also be necessary for this type of swimmer to take more of a lifting breath than is usually desirable. They may also find they need to swim with the pull buoy to compensate for their body drag.

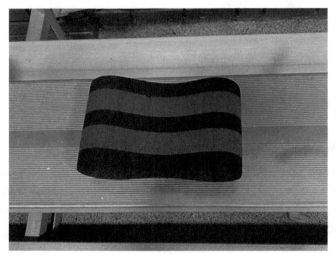

*Pull buoy.*

## C  Dealing With the Fearful Swimmer

When dealing with the fearful swimmer, the overall lesson plan goes out the window! Initially, it will all be about making the student comfortable in the water. All the swimming steps that have been previously mentioned will be greatly slowed down. Section II on making the student comfortable in the water will still happen in succession but at a much slower pace.

**Be mindful with the fearful student that learning to stand in the water after a push-off from the wall is extremely important.** Until the student has mastered the standing motion, they will remain fearful in the water. Once they know how to stand in the water, the fear will still be there but at a greatly reduced level.

With the fearful swimmer, it may be advisable to have them use a waist aqua belt or a life vest, but do so on a limited basis, as it can become a crutch for the student, and they will become reluctant to get into the water without it.

When teaching the standing method to the fearful swimmer, the water barbell becomes very important and helpful. First, it will help the student with their kicking motion, and it makes it easier to do the pulling-your-arms-to-your-chest sequence, as they can physically pull down on the barbell and get themselves into the proper position.

Dealing with the fearful swimmer will call for a great deal of patience—I have had students who needed six or seven lessons to master the standing motion. Also, if there are any gaps in lessons with a fearful swimmer, there can be a significant amount of regression as they return to their fearful state. Be sure to say encouraging words about their progress, no matter how small that progress may be. Point out to the student that they are now trying to push off from the wall and stand, whereas in the first lesson, they were hesitant to put their face in the water.

## D  Bad Tempo and Pawing the Water

Now is a good time to demonstrate to your swimmer the difference between an effective stroke versus an ineffective one. Tell the student that it is a matter of the splashers versus the non-splashers.

Show the student what bad form looks like—swim a few strokes while thrashing around in the water with a great deal of splashing. Next demonstrate a smooth, efficient stroke. Ask the student which stroke would be better for a workout? Point out to the student that while it is possible for the thrasher to swim, you rarely see them swim a full lap and a swimming workout is beyond their abilities.

The splashing and thrashing in the water are a result of the swimmer moving their arms too quickly through the water without getting an efficient stroke. They are, in effect, windmilling through the water without the necessary pull-push under the water. This swimmer is "pawing" the water—that is, only grazing the water with their hand and not following through with the stroke. Stand behind the student and show them how to do the stroke by taking their arms through the correct motion. If the swimmer continues to take a shallow stroke, it may be necessary to demonstrate the stroke out of the water by having the student lie on a bench as you show them the proper form.

Show the student someone who swims with their upper body out of the water. Tell the swimmer that it is possible to swim that way and never put their face in the water, but that person also has very limited swimming abilities and tires very quickly.

Tell the student to observe swimmers in the pool and notice who splashes when they swim and who does not—the difference will certainly be what you have demonstrated to them.

But if your student continues to struggle with any of the problems mentioned above, it may be time to consider something else: **Freestyle is not for everyone!** They may feel more comfortable with a hybrid mix of freestyle and breaststroke and even some "doggie paddle" when breathing. Continue to work with the student until they have achieved a stroke that allows them to take a breath and develop enough stamina to swim a lap.

# PART II
# TEACHING BACKSTROKE

Instructors will find that most students enjoy swimming backstroke. It is much easier to breathe as their face is out of the water.

To start, tell your student that it is very important to tilt their head all the way back, with their chin pointed to the ceiling as far back as they can go. Doing so will throw their shoulder blades back, arching and bowing their back, which brings their feet and legs to the surface. Arms come back, brushing their ears, and the hands enter the water pinky finger first. The arm motion is similar to the freestyle: the arms pull down from the surface until the elbow is parallel with the hip and then the hand snaps down. Both arms must be in constant motion—when one arm is pulling down, the other arm is coming out of the water. At the same time, the legs must be kicking to compensate for the arm strokes.

When first demonstrating the stroke, stand behind the student and position their head correctly by placing your hands under their chin and moving the chin upward to look at the ceiling, and then have the swimmer start to stroke. After they have taken a few strokes, it may be necessary to position your hand on the small of the student's back to bring their lower body to the surface.

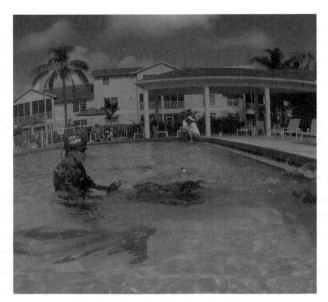

*Backstroke—positioning the head.*

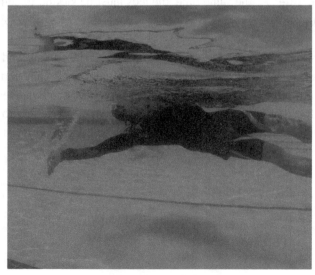

*Backstroke—pull down.*

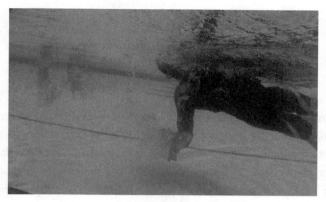

*Backstroke—arm beginning slap down.*

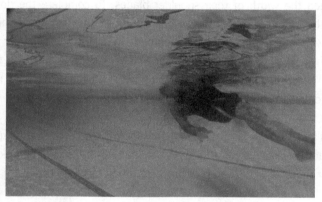

*Backstroke—arm extended after flip down.*

This is a good time to show the swimmer the flags that are strung across the pool at both ends. Advise the student that the flags are there to let a backstroker know that they are approaching the wall. Once your student is comfortable with the stroke, position them just beyond the flags and have them swim toward the wall, counting their strokes as they swim—you will be standing next to the wall ready to stop them with your hand when they get close. Ask the student how many strokes they counted, and then tell them what the total amount of strokes would be to the wall, and once they get to two less than the total, they should look for the wall.

# PART III
# TEACHING BREASTSTROKE

The breaststroke, like treading water, involves two very different motions, which may be difficult for the student to master initially. The arm motion is a pressing down with the hands, like someone pushing themselves out of the pool. That is a good demonstration technique to show the swimmer how much more effective it is to push out of the pool with your arms in front of you rather than taking your arms wide. Tell your student that the arm motion downward should not exceed the width of their shoulder blades. To complete the downward motion the swimmer brings their elbows and forearms together. This is the *chicken wing* motion and when done properly will cause the swimmer to come out of the water, raising their shoulder blades and torso, allowing them to breathe. The downward arm stroke ends with the hands pressed together under the breastbone with the hands together in prayer position.

The arm press-down takes place at the same time as the swimmer's legs come back toward their butt. This is the loading up phase of the kick. The swimmer then sends his hands in prayer position out over the water.

When the arm press-down and *chicken wing* is executed correctly, the swimmer should rise up out of the water clearing their head, shoulder blades, and mid-chest. This is when the student takes their breath. At the same time as the swimmer performs the arm motion, they simultaneously send their legs outward, generating the movement from their hips, and ending with a strong snapping motion of the ankles coming together, rather than the legs moving straight backward from the thighs. The head is placed between the arms with the waterline at mid-forehead while the swimmer exhales. Once the arms are fully extended and the legs have come together, tell the student to allow for a few seconds of glide before starting the next stroke.

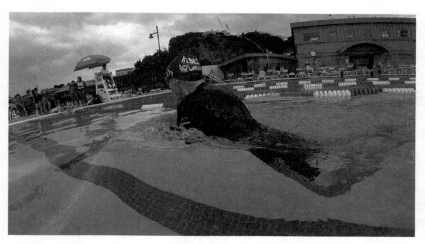

*Breaststroke—arms and legs loading.*

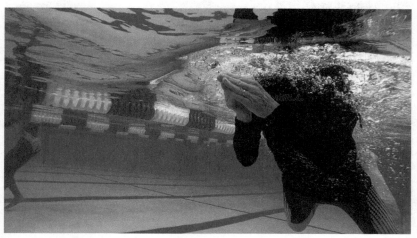

*Breaststroke—arms beginning chicken wing.*

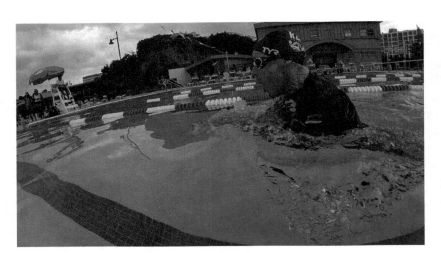

*Breaststroke—chicken wing completed.*

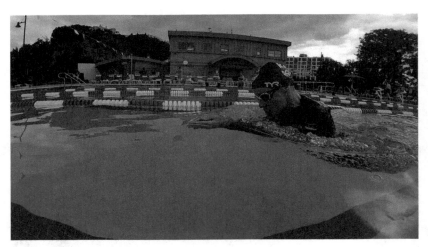

*Breaststroke—arms extending.*

Although the breaststroke is relatively easy for a student to learn, invariably, there are some initial problems. The student will likely bring their hands too wide—well outside the distance of their shoulder blades, which hampers a strong pull-down and *chicken wing* action which hinders forward momentum.

And, as we have mentioned, they will likely kick their legs straight back rather than out to the sides.

Also with the arms and the downward motion, it is very likely that the swimmer will bring their hands too far down and end up with their hands on their thighs instead of under their breastbone.

Another common error will be an inability to synchronize their arms with the kicking motion. To help correct this, have the student hold on to the side as you demonstrate the proper leg kick. As you bring their feet up to their butt, say: "Your arms are coming back," and when you shoot their legs back, you say: "Your hands shoot out." Then demonstrate the stroke for the student. First have them observe you swim as they look above the water. Next demonstrate as they look under the water while you swim by them.

Continue to work with the student until they can synchronize both motions into a smooth stroke. Work with them on the glide at the end of the stroke. Once the student has become proficient in the stroke, teach them how to take their first stroke. When starting from the wall, the first breaststroke motion is performed by pushing off under the water with arms stretched out in front and the head tucked between the arms. After reaching a full glide under the water, the arms are pulled down on either side of the body, at the same time, a dolphin kick (both feet together kicking down and up) is executed (advise the student that elite swimmers take a number of dolphin kicks), and after as many dolphin kicks as the swimmer can manage underwater, the swimmer surfaces and begins stroking.

# PART IV
# TEACHING BUTTERFLY

If your student has successfully mastered freestyle, backstroke, and breaststroke, you may want to finish by teaching them butterfly.

Keep in mind, however, that butterfly is not an easy stroke for the beginner. Like breaststroke, it involves two quite different motions, but the arm stroke takes a good deal of upper body strength, so it is not for everyone.

The arm stroke is performed by using the shoulders to bring the arms around in a rolling action over the water. At the same time, a double dolphin kick is executed, once when the arms start to rotate over the water and again when the hands are entering the water and the arms begin their downward motion, thus helping to propel the arms through the water.

Once the swimmer's arms enter the water, they push down and make an S pattern through the water. As the swimmer is finishing the arm motion at the end of the S pattern arc, they raise their head out of the water to breathe. The swimmer can elect to either breathe by pulling their head up or turning their head to the side. Usually, the forward head motion is considered preferable.

Upon successful completion of the butterfly, your student now knows the entire swimming repertoire.

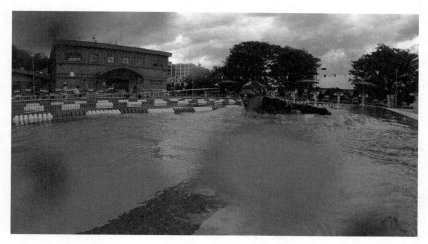

*Butterfly beginning stroke.*

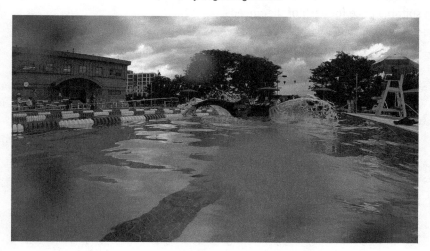

*Butterfly mid-stroke.*

# PART V
# SWIM INSTRUCTION SUMMARY

Teaching swimming calls for a great deal of patience on the part of the instructor. It is also a process of constant observation and evaluation as no two students are ever exactly alike in their ability to respond to lessons. Some students will take to the swimming part of the lessons but have difficulty with treading water, while another student will be the exact opposite. It is also difficult when teaching more than one student at a time as it is extremely rare that two or more students will respond to lessons at the same pace. It is a challenge to the instructor to continue to bring those students along at a suitable pace for each of their needs.

It is also a rare student who will take lessons through the entire process of learning other strokes beyond freestyle. This is understandable as completing the waterproof process of freestyle is often challenging enough. My recommendation is to tell the student (after they have completed the freestyle-waterproofing stage of their development) to work on building up their stamina to the point where they can swim laps and then think about coming back for a refresher course or to start learning the additional strokes—their choice.

**Always be mindful that it is impossible to praise your student too much**. I am always surprised how often a student will dwell on any part of the lesson they are not getting and forget that they are now freely swimming in the water without fear!

At any rate, take pride in the fact that you have given your student a tool that will enhance their life while making them safe in the water.

Well done!

# PART VI
# BUILDING STAMINA AND WORKING OUT

Building stamina goes hand in hand with elevating swimming skills and becoming an intermediate swimmer. It is just a matter of continuing to improve their swimming skills and building their stamina in the pool. As they spend more time in the pool, they will find that swimming a lap becomes easier, and they are becoming less winded with each lap and more efficient in the water.

As the swimmer is now entering the intermediate stage of swimming, it is a good time to begin to refine their stroke from the basic elements of beginner swimming and the more refined elements of technique that will take the swimmer to the next level.

Tell the swimmer they can now try looking down rather than straight out and try having the water level at the crown of their head, rather than mid-forehead. Also instruct them to reach farther with their strokes, extending their arms after their hands have entered the water and reaching from their shoulder blades and, after that full extension, rolling a bit on their sides to cut down on water resistance and further increase their kicking.

This may be a good time to have someone video their strokes at the beginning and end of their workouts to see if any areas need improvement. Remember that, as we have mentioned, less splash usually reflects an improved stroke.

Begin each workout with four head bobs with exhaling. The head bobs will serve two purposes: first, they will test whether their goggles are tight enough or whether they are leaking water. Second, they will start the oxygenation of their respiratory system. It is also a good idea to do head bobs throughout the workout to combat fatigue and maximize circulation and breathing capacity.

Start the workout by having the student do 4 × 25 yards of freestyle and stopping at the end of each lap, being mindful of a different aspect of their stroke with each lap. For instance, on lap 1 have them focus on their arm stroke and whether their elbows are lifting high as they picture taking their elbow to the far end of the pool.

Second lap, they focus on their breathing—are they looking down with the water level at the crown of their head? Are they executing an easy head turn and taking a sip of air and totally exhaling before their next stroke?

Next lap, turn the focus to that iron bar that we talked about that runs through their shoulder blades. Are they pressing their torso slightly down and being mindful that they are stroking with their arms and rotating their rotator cuffs while keeping the rest of their torso stabilized?

On their fourth lap, tell them to let their mind go as they swim freely without concentrating on anything. How did that feel?

We are now ready to begin the workout.

Time the student with the pool clock or a stopwatch while swimming two laps at 75%-80% of their speed capacity. Upon completing the two laps, check their time and how long it takes their breathing to return to normal. Now have them swim another two laps and see if they can maintain the same time interval for the two laps and whether that same rest period is adequate to return their breathing to normal. If not, add 5-10 seconds to the rest period, then try another two laps, noting their swim time and rest period—adding 5 or 10 seconds for the rest as needed.

After four laps of freestyle, have them try two laps of backstroke. Do a similar stroke check as they did with freestyle. In the first lap, tell them be mindful if your nose and chin are pointing back and whether their back is sufficiently bowed. Are their arms entering the water at the 11 and 1 o'clock positions? Are their hands entering the water pinkie first? Now have them swim a second lap with the proper form. If you are satisfied with their form and further stroke correction is not needed, time them for two laps of backstroke at the same 70%–80% of speed. Note the time and the period of rest they need. Repeat another four laps of backstroke using the same method of repeating their swim and rest time.

Once they backstroke segment is complete, it is time to move on to their breaststroke section. Begin with the same mindful stroke check. As we have noted before, the breaststroke involves two very different motions, so their pre-check exam may take longer.

Take a lap breaking down the stroke. Are their hands coming down just under your breastbone? Are they doing the *chicken wing* arm motion with their head and raising their shoulders out of the water? Or, are their hands ending on their thighs?

On the second lap have them concentrate on their kick. Is their kick generating outward or going straight back? Remind them that they want to try and create a frog-like kick motion. Are they loading their kick as their arms come to under their breastbone and sending the kick outward as their arms shoot through the water in a prayer position? Are their movements fully synchronized into two motions, or are they doing the motions independent of each other, which is hindering their forward momentum?

After two laps of stroke evaluation, have them begin swimming four laps using the same time intervals for swimming and resting.

Once they have completed all three strokes, have them take a rest until they are at full recovery. Now, time them for 50 yards in each stroke at the same 75–80% stroke speed when fully rested.

You now have a baseline on which to structure their workouts. Begin to add to the workouts by increasing the number of laps they swim while decreasing the time intervals they take to rest. This will be the same structure you will use on each level of your swimming: beginner, intermediate, and advanced.

# PART VII
# WORKOUTS FOR LIFE—
# INTERMEDIATE LEVEL

These workouts can be given to your students. They are intended to help the swimmer continue to improve and keep swimming for life.

## Ladders

A ladder workout is one that works on all levels of swimming ability. It is also an easy way to quickly accumulate a lot of yardage.

Begin by swimming an easy 500 yards, which will also work as your warm-up. I find it helpful when distance swimming to use a pull buoy (see also Swim Equipment), particularly in the early segments. After the 500 yards, rest until your breathing returns to normal, and then swim 400 yards with the same rest period. Continue to drop each swim amount—300, 200, 100, 50, and then back up to 500. Switch out your strokes at whatever yardage is comfortable for you. You can also do sprints on the smaller lap intervals. At the end of the ladder, you will have swum a total of 3,100 yards. If that amount of yardage is too difficult, begin with a comfortable amount—300 or 200 yards.

## High-Intensity Interval Training: HIIT

Do not fall into the trap of thinking you need a particular amount of time to get in a good workout. Always remember that it is possible to get in a good workout, no matter the amount of time you have in the pool.

A good way to get a good workout in with a limited time amount is through high-intensity interval training, also known as HIIT.

Swim 400 or 500 yards as a warm-up. The rest of the workout is under the clock. Time yourself for 100 yards/meters at a sprint level. You want your swim to be fast but at a pace where you can duplicate that time repeatedly. Take note of that time and use it as a baseline. Take a rest that allows you to return close to normal breathing. My "go to" set has been 100 yards every 2 minutes.

Do as many repeat intervals that are comfortable while maintaining that first time. You will find this varies depending on how you are feeling that day. I try to do anywhere from 3-5 intervals of 100 yards on 2 minutes and then an easy 50-100 yards, and then repeat the intervals.

As I've said, if you only have half an hour to swim, this is an excellent workout.

# PART VIII
# SWIM EQUIPMENT

## Pull Buoys

As I have mentioned, I am a big advocate of pull buoys. I find that the plaining-off motion that they help create makes my swims much more comfortable and allows me to swim further with less expenditure of effort—and who doesn't want that?

In addition, pull buoys are also extremely helpful for teaching freestyle and, as previously mentioned, very helpful for the student who drags their lower body.

When using a pull buoy the lower-body draggers almost always note the difference between how their body is positioned on top of the water from how their body is positioned when they swim without the pull buoy. After using the pull buoy tell the student, "That is how you want your body to be positioned when you swim." You can also encourage them to use a pull buoy when working out and practicing their stroke.

## Hand Paddles

Many swimmers like to couple swim buoys with hand paddles. There are pros and cons to using hand paddles. On the plus side, they encourage a proper pull technique and strong follow-through. On the negative side, a hand paddle, because it creates a maximized pull, also creates a lot of torque and stress on the shoulders and rotator cuffs. Swimmers are prone to shoulder injuries, particularly as they age. Therefore, it may be best to use hand paddles initially on a limited basis to see how your body reacts to them.

There are different types of hand paddles—some are flat and have rubber or plastic straps that your fingers slip into. Another type is a glove in which your hands are completely enclosed.

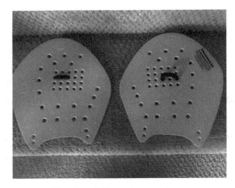

*Hand paddles—strap-on type.*

## Kickboards

Kickboards are an essential tool for working on your kicking form. They are also a good way to break up your swim workout by interspersing some kicking drills. Be mindful while kicking with a kickboard that the upward kick is as important as the downward kick. Remember that the downward kick is generated by the hips, whereas the upward kick is generated by the thighs.

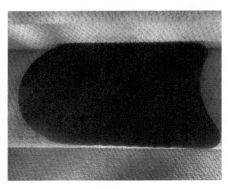

*Kickboard.*

# Flippers

Flippers are an excellent addition to your workout and are also very versatile. They can be used while kicking with kickboards or to supplement your strokes. Some swimmers who struggle with kicking and using a kickboard find their kicking is greatly enhanced by using flippers.

In addition, flippers can be a real asset while doing other strokes, such as butterfly. They also can help with breaking up your workout by interspersing some kicking drills or swimming some sets with the fins.

Try doing a set of individual medleys (butterfly, backstroke, breaststroke, freestyle) while wearing flippers. Then do some kicking laps, and then go back to the individual medley sets.

Flippers can also break up workouts by doing some sprinting sets of 25s or 50s. I am a big advocate of really trying to elevate your heart rate during a swim workout, and there is no better way to do that than by sprinting for a part of your workout.

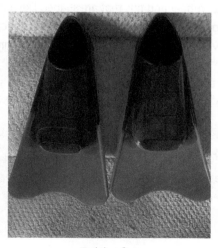

*Training fins.*

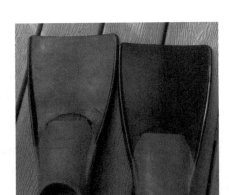

*Flipper-long fins.*

As with hand paddles, there are different types of flippers. There are small flippers that have very small fins and are made with a hard plastic or rubber shell and geared just for swim workouts. There are also flippers with long fins and made with softer rubber and fins that are shaped like a fish tail and made strictly for working out. The fish tail type of swim fins is difficult to make turns with and would only be recommended for experienced swimmers.

Just be careful not to buy the swim fins that are made for scuba diving and divers as those are made with a heavy, thick rubber that is unsuitable for swim workouts.

As I grew older, I found that the small fins were hard on my calf muscles and often gave me cramps (a common problem for older swimmers), and I switched to a longer fin style.

## Snorkels

Snorkels are excellent tools to assist the swimmer with concentrating and focusing on their pulling or kicking technique. Also, they are helpful for swimmers who struggle with breathing. Just take care not to rely on the snorkel too much, which can come at the expense of your breathing technique.

We are talking about the snorkels that are made for swimmers rather the type that is geared toward recreational snorkeling or scuba.

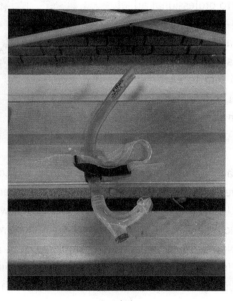

*Snorkel.*

# ABOUT THE AUTHOR

**Coach Brian "Flash" Fagan** has taught and coached swimming for over 30 years. He has taught swimming to all age groups, from infants to adults in their 70s and 80s. He has coached all skill levels, from age group swimmers to professional athletes.

Coach Brian has specialized in swim lessons for adults who were fearful in the water, which led him to evolve his Flash Aquatic Swim Technique that significantly breaks away from how swimming has been taught to adults over the last 50 years.

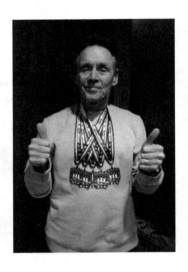

Coach Brian was a New York State swim champion in high school and an NCAA division II swimmer. He was a New York State Jones Beach and Robert Moses State Park Ocean Lifeguard for 13 years. He is a US Masters Swimming Certified Adult Swim Instructor and a US Masters Swimming certified swim coach level II. He is a 22-time New Jersey Masters swim champion. Coach Brian is currently the Adult Swim Instruction Director at the Rutherford Swim Association in Rutherford, New Jersey. He is the Owner and Founder of Flash Aquatics.

He lives in Lincoln Park, New Jersey, and Sarasota, Florida, with his wife Renee.

Contact Coach Brian through brianflashaqua@gmail.com, CoachBrianFagan@LinkedIn.com, or Brian@RutherfordSwim.org.

*What students have said about the FLASH AQUATICS swimming technique. They reference the fact that they became "Waterproof", meaning they were able to jump into the deep end of the pool—12 feet—come to the surface and tread water, and then swim 25 meters, something that less than 25% of the adult population in America can do.*

Coach Brian gives me a challenge and a sense of accomplishment through swimming. I had such a great experience of overcoming my fear of deep water through Brian's swimming class. I am looking forward to classes with him in the future. Brian, thank you for teaching me to swim.

—Nael B.K., 55

With Coach Brian's swim technique, I was comfortable swimming in just three lessons and waterproof after six! Learning to swim has been on my bucket list for years. I am happy to have finally learned to swim thanks to Coach Brian.

—Matt J., 38

I had an incredible experience with Brian as my swim coach. In just six lessons I went from barely knowing how to swim to feeling confident and being waterproof. I highly recommend his technique for anyone looking to improve their swimming skills.

—Josephine M., 32

I had an extreme fear of the water due to a traumatizing experience as a child which caused me to delay swimming lessons until I was 28 years old. Coach Brian helped me overcome my fears of swimming by teaching me not only to swim but to love the water in every situation. I was able to cliff dive and scuba dive in Bali after just eight lessons.

—Lilly L., 28

**Credits**

Cover and interior design:  Anja Elsen
Layout:  DiTech Publishing Services, www.ditechpubs.com
Cover photo:  © AdobeStock
Interior photos:  Courtesy of Brian Fagan
Managing editor:  Elizabeth Evans
Copy editor:  Sarah Tomblin, www.sarahtomblinediting.com

# SWIM WITH MEYER & MEYER SPORT

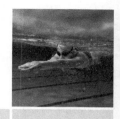

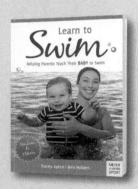

$9.95 US
ISBN: 9781782551607

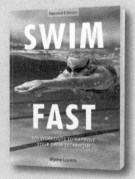

$16.95 US
ISBN: 9781782552604

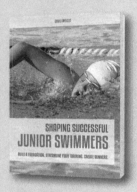

$19.95 US
ISBN: 9781782551409

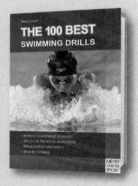

$19.95 US
ISBN: 9781841263373

| | | |
|---|---|---|
| **MEYER & MEYER Sport** | Phone | +49 02 41 - 9 58 10 - 13 |
| Von-Coels-Str. 390 | Fax | +49 02 41 - 9 58 10 - 10 |
| 52080 Aachen | E-Mail | sales@m-m-sports.com |
| Germany | Website | www.m-m-sports.com |

MEYER
& MEYER
SPORT